STRESS BUSTER

HOW TO LIVE A STRESS FREE LIFE IN A STRESSFUL ENVIRONMENT

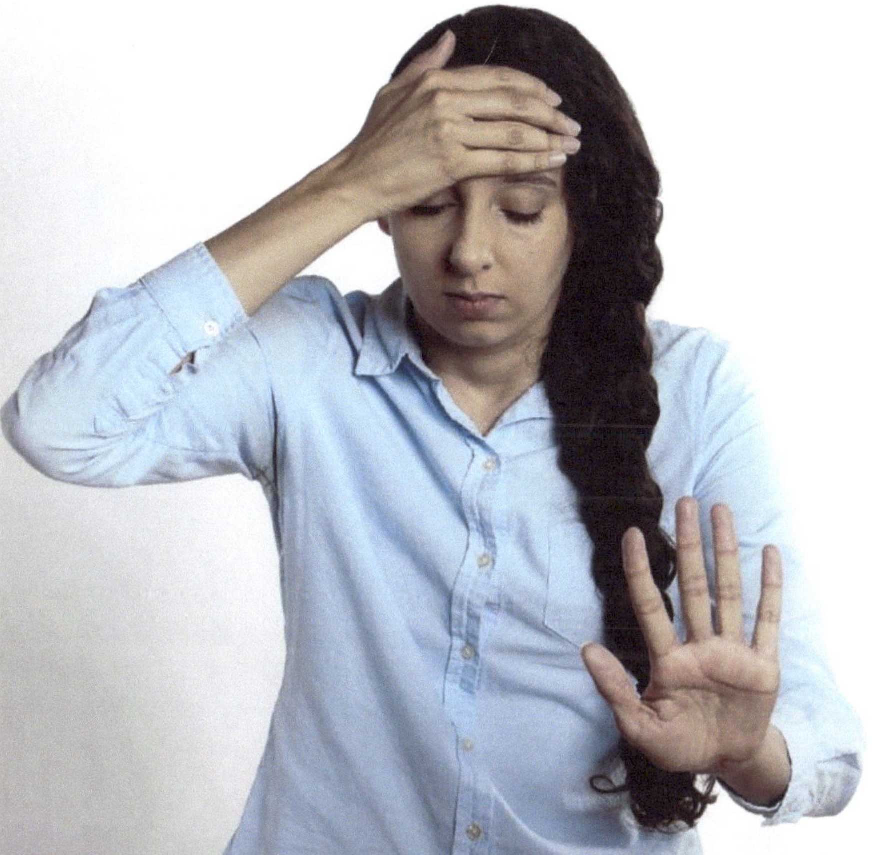

ADENIJI JAMIU

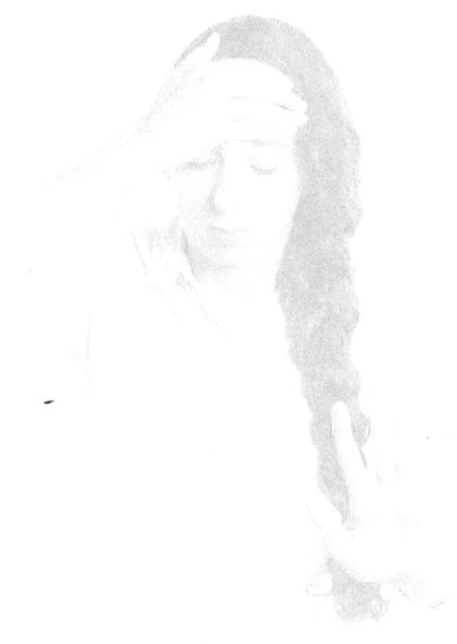

ACKNOWLEDGEMENT

I give glory and adorations to Almighty God, the omniscience, omnipresence. The giver and taker of life. The Alpha and Omega. The owner and controller of the Universe. Who gave us life and purpose for life.

I will through God thank my both parents whom God used as the vessel that convey me to this world.

My profound gratitude goes and not limited to (in no particular order of ranking):

Coach Edirin Edewor who's been the main motivator indirectly towards the success of this master piece. A great mindset coach and a 2 times Amazon bestseller. You want to write your book and get it published in less than 7 days? Then hook her up.

Odunayo Oludele (my other half). She is the first lady I ever met in my life that supports my dream and aspirations. She knows I'm crazy for success and she supports every aspect of the journey. With you, 2017 was one of the best and greatest year of my life.

Wisdom Bradford--- my graphic designer. I always thought hiring a graphic designer "online" will be a disaster. Bradford made me experience the opposite of that. I recommend him.

Sesan Kareem (KAS)—Sesan Kareem is an author, a pharmacist, a catalyst for growth and an inspiration for personal fulfillment and lasting result. He is also the team leader and founder of Mareek Image Concepts. You are one of the great motivator and mentor I crossed path with this year 2017.

Dr. Ifeanyi Atueyi—Dr. Ifeanyi is the Publisher and Managing Director of Phamanews – West Africa's foremost health journal. He is an icon of pharmacy. The idea of this book was birthed when I attended one of his trainings on " Stress Management and Healthy Living."

I also want to give a big shout out to all members of Online Publishers and Entrepreneurs Network (OPEN) a Facebook community of writers as well as entrepreneurs of different spheres of life. Thank you all for your unrelenting efforts in pushing and dragging (if need be) one another to succeed. You guys are really amazing and are the real MVPs.

I might be an ingrate if I forget to acknowledge Dr. Besh Ladi (first buyer of this book) for believing in me to order for this book about 30 minutes of announcing the "pre-order" of it.

Finally I say a big thank you to all and sundry.

My wish for you is a "Stress free Long Life."

God bless you all.

TABLE OF CONTENTS

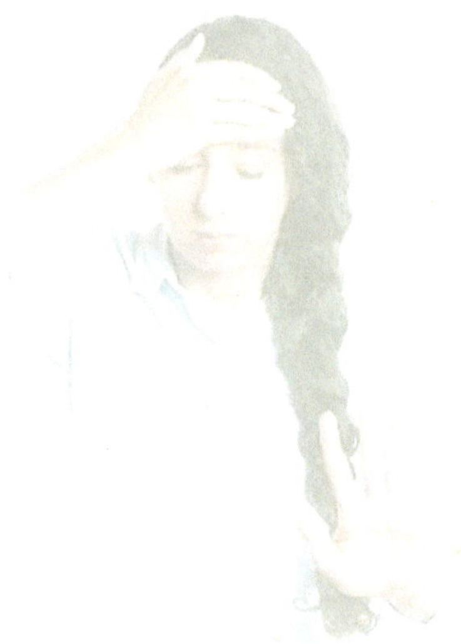

INTRODUCTION

Dear friend,

Thank you for buying this book.

The fact that you bought this book shows that you want to live a professional/personal stress free life even if you found yourself in a stressful environment (which is inescapable). You want people to emulate your healthy stress free lifestyle. You are two steps away from it. One, reading this book and two, following through with the techniques taught in this book.

Stress can be a real deadly omen that can ever happen to us, both in our personal and professional lives.

The fact that we are in one of the most technologically advanced time in the history of mankind (which will increase) has been a major contributor to increase in stress.

The purpose of this book is to teach you what to do to manage stress in order to live a long stress free happy life.

The Stress Buster is the perfect solution for busy entrepreneurs, managers, professionals as well as individuals who desire to live a healthy "stress free" long life.

In this book (The Stress Buster), you are going to learn step by step guides on stress management without spending a dime on drugs that will eventually do more harm than good.

The STRESS BUSTER in your hands, stress in the grave.

CHAPTER ONE

WHAT IS STRESS?

Stress as the name implies is a very deep and wide topic to cover.

However, for the purpose of this book, we'd familiarize ourselves with the meaning of STRESS as follows:

Stress is primarily a physical response. When stressed, the body thinks it is under attack and switches to "fight or flight" mode, releasing a complex mix of hormones and chemicals such as adrenaline, cortisol, and norepinephrine to prepare the body for physical action.

Stress is the reaction to excessive pressures. Stress arises when people worries that they can't cope with the pressures.

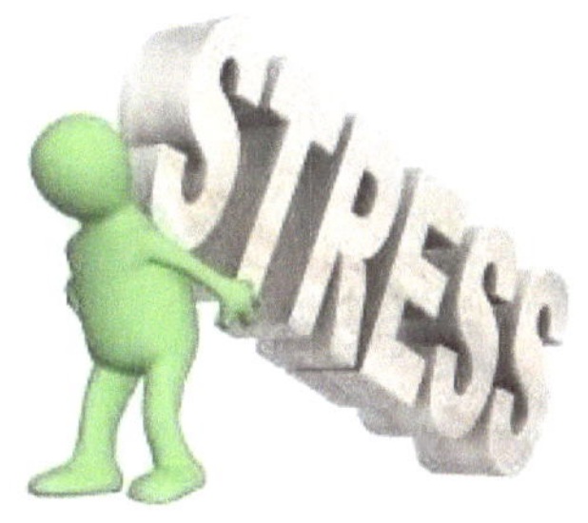

Stress also occurs when the pressure is greater than the resources to cope with the elements causing it.

In a layman term, stress is the wear and tear of the body systems due to usage, aging, and undue expectations & aspirations.

To generalize what stress is, we say," stress is anything that disturbs our mental, mind, emotional, economic and physical equilibrium.

When the stability of any of these is disrupted, then problem surfaces.

However, no matter how or what we define stress as, it always varies from individual to individual. This means that what stresses Mr A might not stress Mr B.

For example, going swimming might be stressful to some, but for others, it might be enjoyable.

In the next chapter, you will learn FORMS OF STRESS.

CHAPTER TWO

FORM OF STRESS

Stress can be GOOD or BAD.

When used correctly, stress releases hidden reserves of creative energy. This insinuates that you must be stressed in order to do something "phenomenal." Otherwise, you're in your comfort zone (where you're not supposed to be).

This is otherwise known as "GOOD" stress (Eustress).

Meanwhile when there's little stress, you feel bored, and no motivation to do anything.

Too much stress on the other hand produces anxiety, worry, confusion and zapping of self confidence.

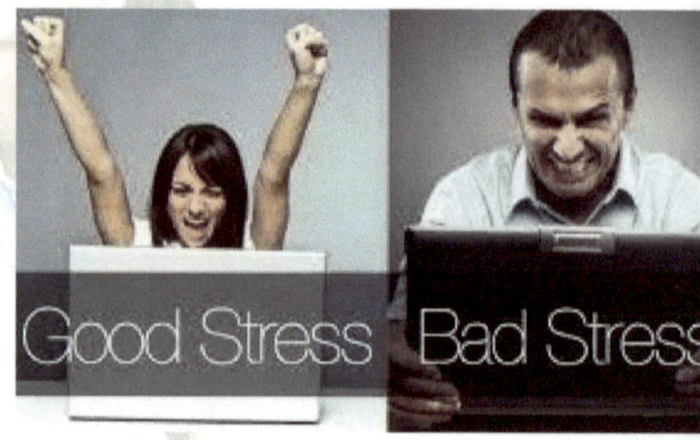

This is otherwise known as "BAD" stress (Distress).

Although we need stress to keep us going on our day-to-day activities, but excess of it is bad.

In the next chapter, you will learn TYPES OF STRESS.

CHAPTER THREE

TYPES OF STRESS

Although according to research, there are different school of thought on stress;

A school of thought believed there are 7 types of stress, another believed it to be 4.

However, the most acceptable and known type of stress is 3.

There are 3 types of stress namely; Acute, Episodic Acute, and Chronic.

1. Acute Stress: This is the most common type of stress. It is the body immediate reaction to a new challenge, event or demand, and it triggers the 'fight or flight' response.

Example of this is an argument with a family member, a costly mistake at work, a near-miss automobile accident, severe acute stress such as stress suffered as the victim of a crime or life-threatening situation which can lead to mental health problems like posttraumatic stress disorder or acute stress disorder.

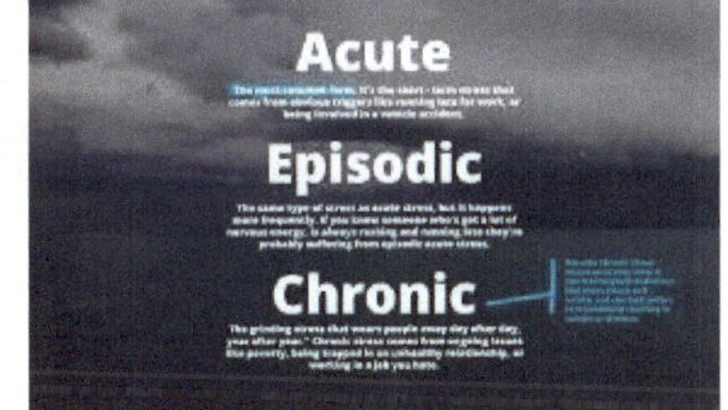

2. Episodic Acute Stress: As it sounds, Episodic acute stress occurs when Acute stress happens frequently.

People who always seem to be having a crisis tend to have Episodic Acute Stress. They are often short-tempered, irritable, and anxious.

Negative health effects are persistent in their lifestyle, as they accept stress as a part of life.

3. Chronic Stress: If Acute Stress isn't resolved and begins to increase or lasts for long periods of time, it becomes Chronic Stress. This stress is constant and doesn't go away.

This is the stage stress gets to that can make it detrimental to health and cause/contribute to several serious diseases or health risks like; heart attack/disease, accidents, cancer, or even suicide.

In the next chapter, you will learn STRESS MANIFESTATION (SYMPTOMS).

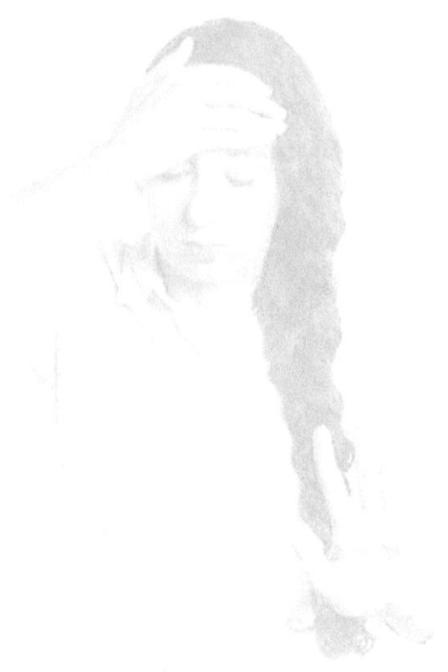

CHAPTER FOUR

STRESS MANIFESTATION (SYMPTOMS)

As we know that symptom is an indication of a disease or disorder that is noticed by the sufferer.

Stress can affect all aspects of life, including emotions, behaviors, thinking ability and physical health.

However, since people handle stress differently, symptoms of stress can vary.

For the purpose of this book, we shall break down stress symptoms into (4) four namely; EMOTIONAL, PHYSICAL, BEHAVIOURAL, & COGNITIVE

Emotional Symptoms of stress include:

- ✓ Feeling bad about oneself (low self esteem).
- ✓ Feeling lonely or worthless
- ✓ Feeling overwhelmed.
- ✓ Having difficulty relaxing.
- ✓ Becoming easily agitated.

2. Physical Symptoms of stress include:

- ✓ Low energy
- ✓ Chest pain
- ✓ Headaches
- ✓ Frequent cold and infection
- ✓ Dry mouth
- ✓ Grinding teeth
- ✓ Loss of sexual desire

3. Behavioral Symptoms of stress include:

- ✓ Increased use of alcohol, drugs and cigarettes
- ✓ Exhibiting nervous behaviors such as nail biting...agbaya..lol.
- ✓ Changes in appetite --- either not eating or eating too much

✓ Avoiding responsibilities

4. Cognitive Symptoms of stress include:

✓ Inability to focus
✓ Being pessimistic
✓ Constant worry
✓ Forgetfulness and disorganization
✓ Racing thoughts

PS: What can bring stress to one person might not bring stress to another depending on the reception.

In the next chapter, you will learn the STRESS REACTION.

CHAPTER FIVE

STRESS REACTION

Having examined the STRESS MANIFESTATION/SYMPTOMS, it is crucial we know how stress come about; How our body systems react that makes us know that we are stressed.

This is not new, we tend to know when we are worked out/off/up or stressed... Don't we?

That's right, we do.......

So, what we want to do here is to know how our body systems work prior and when stressed as well as what happens.

- ✓ Activating events causes changes to occur in the brain. Before stress sets in, certain events triggers the stress hormones.

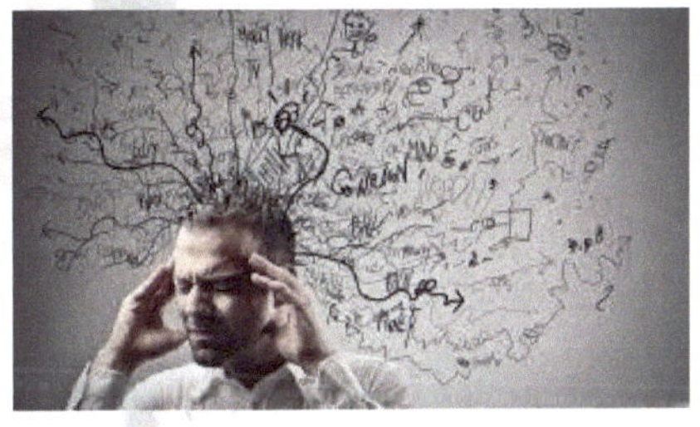

For example (as a banker), you're having a blissful day in the office crunching your goals/targets joyously.

You've been overwhelmed with everything when all of a sudden you remembered you just debited a huge amount you were supposed to credit.

I bet you know what that spells out.......

You'd forget about the excitement you've been having for the past few hours....

End result?... STRESS...

Hope you've not been carried away by the story.... We were looking at the Stress Reaction.

For us to have that result "stress", stage one had come into play. Go back and read it.

- ✓ Stress hormones (adrenaline, cortisol, dopamine seratonin) are released into the blood which brings about complex reaction to the brain.
- ✓ These stress hormones start to affect all parts of the internal organs and systems such as heart (the heart pumps abnormally), livers, kidneys, genitals, muscles etc. This in turn can lead to loss of appetite for sex, urinating less or more.

Little wonder one of the major symptoms of stress is "depression."

Once one, two or all of the above organs/systems is/are affected, the body automatically switches to "flight or fight" mode.

- ✓ The stressed individual tries hard to adapt to the pressures on the organs of the body. Some succeed and some fail.

Let's visit our example again. The "banker" could either adapt to and overcome the stress by forcing himself to correct his mistakes (fight mode), thereby completing his task joyously for the day.

Or he could choose to let the STRESS overpower him and leave him vulnerable for the rest of the day (flight mode).

- ✓ If stress persists, resources gradually become depleted and individual becomes mentally exhausted.

In a situation whereby (the banker) chooses the "flight mode" over the "fight mode," this reaction stage sets in.

- ✓ This is the last and crucial stage of Stress Reaction.

Productivity is affected, immune system is compromised, mental faculty is affected, and stress-related diseases set in.

Stress can really make you look 30 years older than your real age. In the next chapter, you will learn CAUSES OF STRESS.

CHAPTER SIX

CAUSES OF STRESS

We've understood what stress is and what it's not. We've also studied its TYPES, MANIFESTATION(SYMPTOMS) as well as its REACTION.

Therefore, it is crucial we learn its causes too.....

There is no limit to what can cause stress. This means that stress causing agents are so numerous than meet the eyes.

However, we are going to examine some major causes of stress that we don't really pay attention to.

ENVIRONMENTAL CAUSES

The type of environment we live in has a lot to do with our healthy/unhealthy living.

Environment is a great contributor to "how well" organisms (humans) live healthily in their habitat.

The following are environmental stress contributors

- ➢ Noisy environment: Although human respond to stress in different ways, there are those (including myself) who find it difficult to concentrate in a noisy environment.

- ➢ Poor lighting: I personally don't feel comfortable reading under a normal (yellow) bulb. I prefer to use (AKT white) bulb.

- ➢ Hot or cold offices: I can mention a few people I know that don't like staying too long in the banking hall because.....you know the end of the story na.....don't claim "saint" please......

- ➢ Heavy rainfall and flood: we all know heavy rainfall and flood could cause serious damages if not loss of lives which will eventually lead to stress. Take the (Tsunami) case as example.

- ➢ Air pollution

- ➢ Fire disasters
- ➢ Water pollution
- ➢ Building collapses.

SOCIAL/ECONOMIC CAUSES

- ➢ Insecurity { armed robbery, kidnapping even adultnapping....lol...
- ➢ Declining business turn over and profits
- ➢ Fraud (cybercrime)
- ➢ Wickedness/immorality –rape, murder, human trafficking
- ➢ Inflation—rising costs of essential commodities
- ➢ Poor infrastructure – erratic power supply, inadequate water supply, bad roads
- ➢ Unemployment.

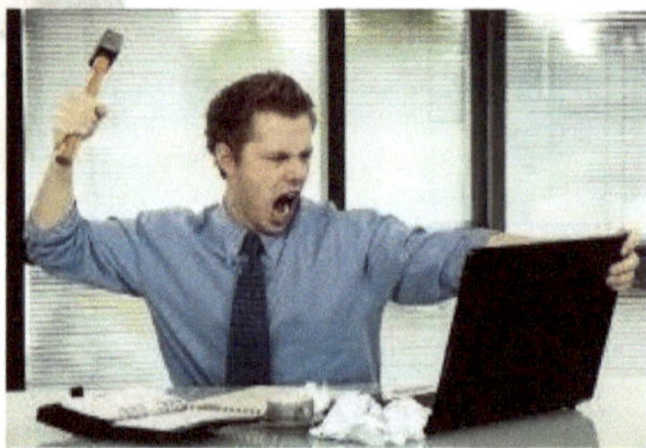

ORGANISATIONAL

- ➢ Office politics – promotion, succession
- ➢ Poor communication skills causing misunderstanding
- ➢ Poor interpersonal relationships
- ➢ Meeting deadlines
- ➢ Job insecurity
- ➢ Poor, irregular or delayed salaries (I used to be a victim of this)
- ➢ Heavy workload/ extended hours of work

LIFE EVENTS

There are so many life events happening to/around us almost on a daily basis which triggers stress (either good or bad)

In the course of this study, We'd divide these life events into two namely; Negative and Positive Life Events.

NEGATIVE

- Loss of job
- Divorce/separation
- Reversal of fortune (MMM)
- Life threatening illness
- Loss of money (stock market)

POSITIVE

- Pregnancy
- Getting married
- Child birth
- Retirement

DAILY HASSLES

- Insecurity of life and property
- Traffic holdups/ lateness to work/late coming from work
- Bad or rough drivers
- Commuting to and from work
- Inadequate rest/sleep
- Vehicle breakdown

NEGATIVE SELF-TALK

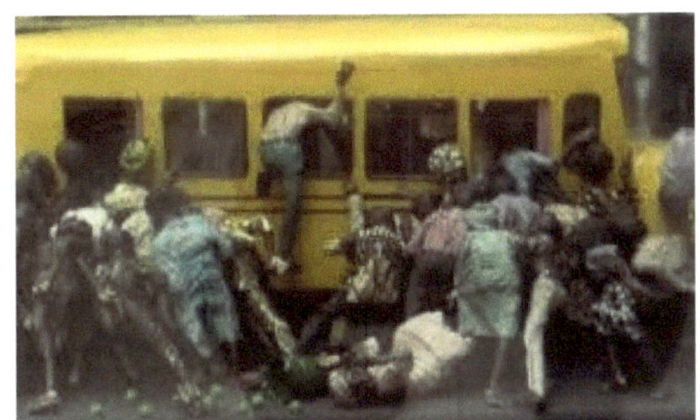

- ➢ Poor intra-personal self-communication

- ➢ Pessimism

- ➢ Self-criticism

- ➢ Reduced self-confidence

- ➢ Poor self-worthiness

- ➢ Seeking for approval

In the next chapter, you will learn HEALTH IMPLICATION OF STRESS.

CHAPTER SEVEN

HEALTH IMPLICATIONS

Stress had been known to be for the aged. However, the story has changed, as survey reveals that millennial aged 18-33 (productive years) are now the most stressful people on earth.

60 to 80% of modern diseases are caused by stress. These diseases include but not limited to;

√ Headache
√ Asthma
√ High blood pressure
√ Heart attack
√ Stroke
√ Infertility (male & female)
√ Insomnia
√ Dementia
√ Obesity
√ Depression
√ Cancer
√ Gastrointestinal problems
√ Premature aging etc

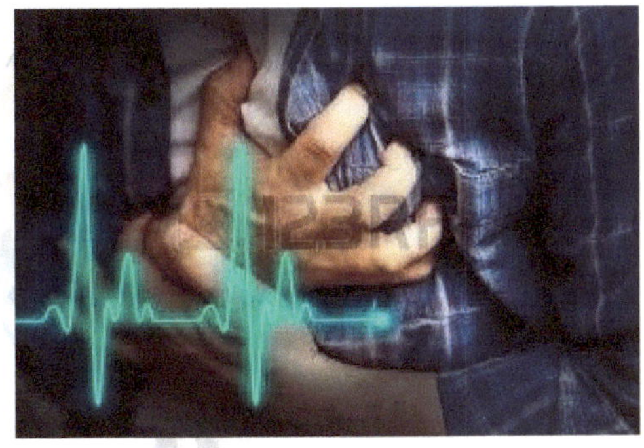

In the next chapter, you will learn STRESS MANAGEMENT TECHNIQUES (how to manage stress).

CHAPTER EIGHT

HOW TO MANAGE STRESS

Having learnt what stress is and what it's not, the TYPES, REACTIONS, MANIFESTATION, CAUSES & IMPLICATION.

We are now on the most important aspect of this book which is STRESS MANAGEMENT (how to manage stress and live stress free in a stressful environment).

And I hope you'd make the most of this......

Let's dive in.........

In order to manage stress, there are many things we need to imbibe.

However, the major aspect to work on if you really desire to live (bad) stress free all day, week, month, year, life long and not spend your hard earned money on drugs that's eventually going to lead you to more complicated health issues later is *DISCIPLINE.*

Yes, you read that word right. You see, all the processes I will be going through here with you involves 99% of your physical participation, hence the need for SELF DISCIPLINE.

However, if you think you'd prefer to spend money to maintain your stress, please feel free to stop reading this material right now......it's not too late yet.

I bet you did not buy it just to read half of it and dump.

Continue reading….

But if you're really tired of spending money you could invest to make more money on stress that you can maintain yourself, then stick with me on this material like ant to sugar.

The processes to managing stress include:

EXERCISE

As we all know that regular exercise burns calories. However, there is more to the madness as exercise not only burn calories. It also burns stress chemicals.

Exercises like; walking, mild jogging, slow deep breathing stimulates the lymphatic system.

DIET

Hippocrate the great father of medicine certainly made us understand that "if the diet is good, medicine is of no need. If the diet is bad, medicine is of no use."

This is to say that we should let medicine be our food and let food be our medicine....(don't misquote please...). In other words, we are to be very mindful and careful of what we eat....

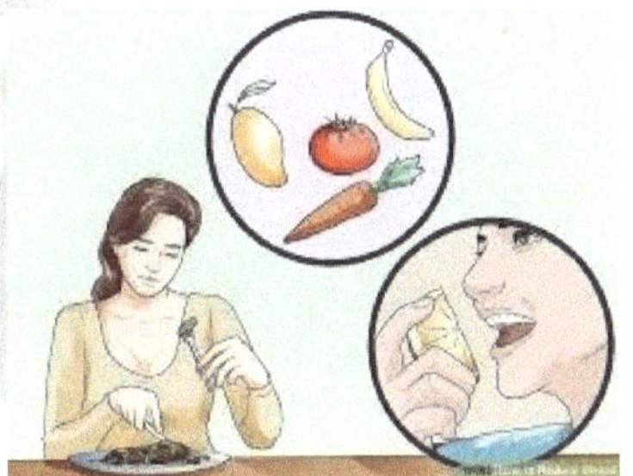

We should avoid:
• Eating food with poor nutritional content--junk, unbalanced diet.

• Eating at the wrong time.

• Rushing the food.

And yes, you must discipline yourself if you really want to achieve that......I can't pamper you....

We've talked about diet and exercise.

Here are the other stress management techniques.....

NEGATIVE NEWS

- Lower your response to negative news from the media. Bad events make news mostly.

- Avoid horrible news and pictures

LEARN TO SMILE AND LAUGH

- Laughter is the best medicine

- Always laugh when you can. It is the cheapest medicine ever.

- "A merry heart doeth good like medicine: but a broken heart drieth the bone." -- Proverbs 17:22

Little wonder, "it takes more muscles to frown than to smile."

STOP TALKING DOWN YOURSELF

- Say positive, confidence- boosting things to yourself.

- Say to yourself always, "Everyday, in every way, I am getting better and better."

  Stop reading this material and say that 5 times…..

  Done?.......

  Good. Continue reading….

- When you do well, congratulate/celebrate yourself (reward yourself)

- When you blunder, look for any good points in what you did as well as the mistakes.

CHANGE YOUR VIEWPOINTS

- Refuse to allow others to stress you. View rudeness or sarcasm as personality defects which are their problem rather than a reflection on your own person.

- Never bear grudges. Forgive your enemies.

- Say something nice to others…..compliment others……

PUT YOUR PROBLEMS INTO PERSPECTIVE

- Be certain that everybody has a problem. The rich also cry. Few problems are truly catastrophic

- Break your problems into smaller ones and solve them one at a time.

- Regard mistakes and set-backs as opportunities to learn. Always try to discover something good in whatever happens to you, no matter how bad it appears at first sight.

- "And we know that all things work together for good to them that love God, to them who are the called according to His purpose."--Romans 8:28

SLOW DOWN

- Stay alone in a quiet room for some minutes and try to remain perfectly still.

- Meditate and reflect on positive thoughts.

- Think on God's blessings and give Him thanks.

BREATHING EXERCISE

- When you become stressed, breathing gets faster and shallower so that only the upper portion of the lungs are used. This produces distressing symptoms that include rapid heartbeat, chest pains, dizziness, anxiety and inability to concentrate.

Try deep, stress reducing breathing as follows:

    ✓ Sit comfortably upright and close your eyes.

- ✓ Place your right hand on your chest and the left on your stomach.

- ✓ Breath in slowly and deeply through your nose.

- ✓ As you exhale, consciously pull in your abdominal muscles using your hand to push down your stomach.

- ✓ Repeat several times.

MANAGE YOUR TIME AND WORK

- Know your biological rhythms.

- Schedule your task to prime time for peak performance.

- Spend adequate time to plan your day.

- Distinguish between urgent and important activities.

- Set SMART (Specific Motivational, Attainable Relevant Trackable) goals.

- Learn to say no without feeling guilty.

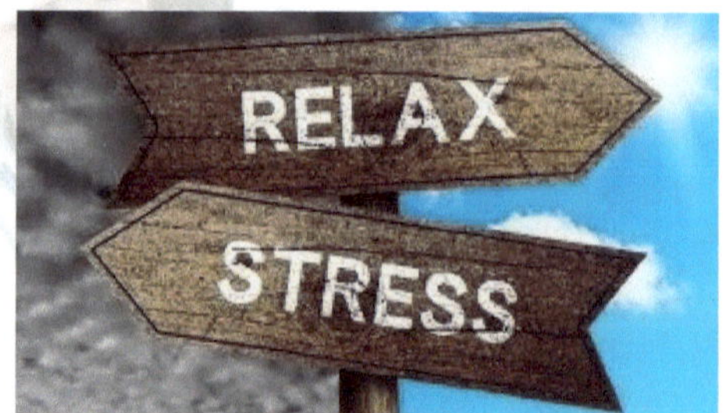

- Don't take more than you can handle.

- Face one task at a time. Don't handle many things at the same time (multitasking)

STOP WORRYING

- "Be anxious for nothing, but in everything by prayer and supplication with thanksgiving let your requests be known to God." --Phil 4:6

- Most of the things we worry about never happen or are beyond our power to control.

- "Come unto me, all ye that labour and are heavy laden, and I will give you rest." --Matt 11:28

CONCLUSION

"The difference between the successful and the failure is action."

Thank you for buying and reading this book. (I hope you didn't miss any point? If you do, go back and read it).

I've shared the techniques that have worked and still working for me, and many other professionals/ experts in their various fields, but no one can help you more than yourself. If you want a change, then you must act. Know that, "if it will be, it is up to YOU."

You have invested by buying and reading this book. Thank you, but all of this will amount to nothing if you do not take any action or use the lessons learned. I bet the techniques shared are easy and costs next to nothing to achieve.

Now, pick up yourself and go live that stress free life you deserved.

To your "stress free" successful living,

Cheers!

About the Author

Adeniji Jamiu is a motivational/public speaker.

He helps smart career individuals build a full or part-time business through network marketing. He's also a health and wellness coach.

He always introduces himself as follows:

I'm Adeniji Jamiu, from Oyo state Nigeria, ready and committed to a successful Tiens business.

Before I joined Tiens, I was a formal educator….. I still educate though…. Yes, I'm a financial educator…………

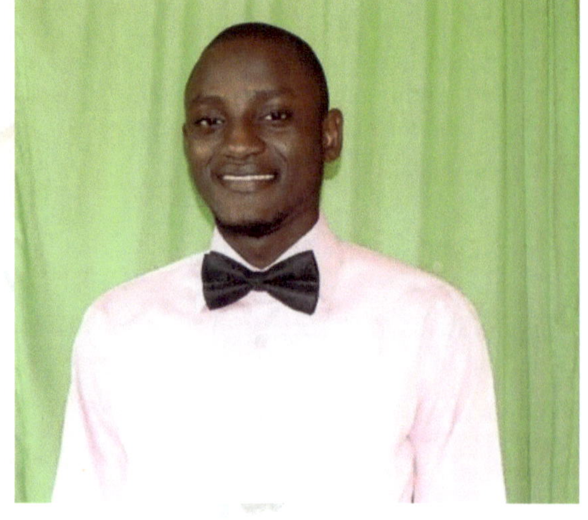

I joined Tiens because I want to live a health and wealthy "stress free" life and to contribute my quota to the development of the world.

My dreams and target is to become a multimillionaire before the age of 35…(guess my age…lol) and to help at least 20,000 individuals achieve their dreams of becoming financially independent.

Thank you for buying this book. Please remember to leave a review and connect with me on my social media platforms.

Facebook: Adeniji Jamiu Bayonle

Facebook Biz Page: www.facebook.com/tiensyoungachievers/

Facebook Personal Page: www.facebook.com/adenijijamiu6

Website: www.tiensyoungachievers.com.ng